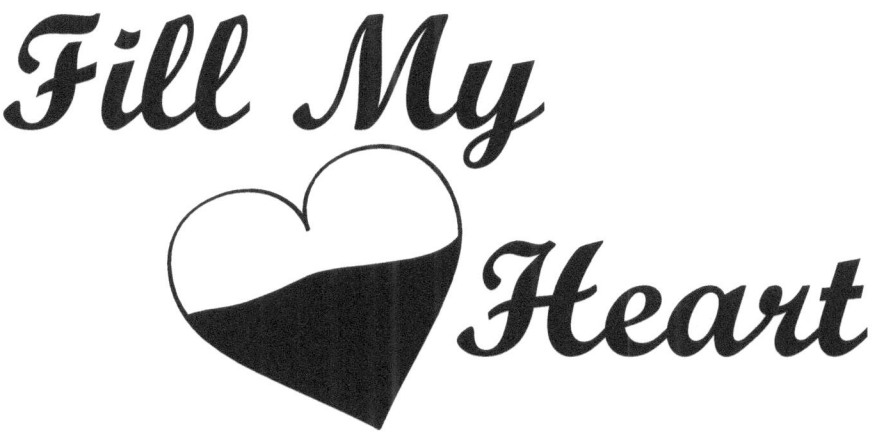

# Fill My Heart

## The Love-Shaped Void Food Was Never Meant to Feed

### by Victoria Lynn Dunn

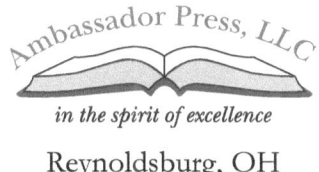

Ambassador Press, LLC
*in the spirit of excellence*
Reynoldsburg, OH

Published by Ambassador Press, LLC
PO Box 722 Reynoldsburg, OH 43068
ambpress@insight.rr.com
www.ambassadorpressllc.com

Copyright © 2008 Victoria Lynn Dunn

Cover Photo © 2008 Curtis Blake
www.curtisblakephotography.com

Cover Design © 2008 Imagine! Studios™
www.artsimagine.com

All rights reserved. No part of this publication may be reproduced or transmitted in any form or by any means, including informational storage and retrieval systems, without permission in writing from the copyright holder, except for brief quotations in a review.

Scripture quotations taken from the 21st Century King James Version®, copyright © 1994. Used by permission of Deuel Enterprises, Inc., Gary, SD 57237. All rights reserved.

Scripture quotations taken from the Amplified® Bible, Copyright © 1954, 1958, 1962, 1964, 1965, 1987 by The Lockman Foundation. Used by permission. (www.Lockman.org)

Scripture quotations taken from the New American Standard Bible®, Copyright © 1960, 1962, 1963, 1968, 1971, 1972, 1973, 1975, 1977, 1995 by The Lockman Foundation
Used by permission. (www.Lockman.org)

ISBN 10: 0-9787850-6-1
ISBN 13: 978-0-9787850-6-2

Library of Congress Control Number: 2008942597

First Ambassador Press, LLC printing, December 2008

# *Dedication*

To the many who've fed my heart and enabled me to feed others—most especially, Virginia Bernice Dunn.

And to my sister, Denise, who fills so many.
Save something for you.

# Foreword by

Apostle Eric L. Warren

# Endorsement by

Susan Ridley

# Foreword

Ecclesiastes 10:10

*If the ax is dull and the man does not whet the edge, he must put forth more strength; but wisdom helps him to succeed.* [Amplified Bible]

In a season when we are inundated with information, impartation becomes all the more significant. I tend to discern the difference between information and impartation based on how I am impacted by the stimulus. Information is good. It leaves me feeling informed, educated, and sometimes equipped. Impartation, on the other hand, changes me. It causes my spirit to leap, my understanding to open, and moves me to act upon that which has stimulated me.

Such is the case with this book, *Fill My Heart*. While Victoria Dunn has penned an excellent story of her personal journey of deliverance from emotional eating, she has captured something more. In the telling of her story, she touches my story and your story and our story: a story based on a fallen world that we all live in, where we all find ourselves clamoring for some sense of significance, affirmation, and identity. In our quest to fit in we take different paths to maintain our equilibrium and continue to feel worthy, worthwhile and significant.

But until we can find the path that leads us to the first thing: our relationship with our maker, we are perpetually frustrated, agitated and unfulfilled. This dissatisfaction leads us into all manner of aberrant living. Some will find temporary but fleeting solace in fashion, some in sports, some in sexual promiscuity, and seriously addictive behaviors, like emotional eating. It all goes back to the same root: We are incomplete and unfulfilled without a genuine abiding relationship with the triune nature of God. The Father, the Son, and the Holy Spirit comprise a spiritual trifecta that heals the hurt, fills in the gaps, and enables us to move beyond pretense to fulfillment of purpose.

Victoria addresses these issues in a unique way that is transparent, revelatory, and moving. As you read this book, you will not only walk with her through her field of dreams, you will travel through your own as well. I have personally never had a weight problem nor any other eating disorder but I recognized the pain; I identified with the struggle, and I rejoiced in the breakthrough because while our "issue" was different, the problem was the same. What is the problem? I'm glad that you asked! The problem is how do we navigate through the storms of life victoriously without having to be something that we are not? And when we find ourselves engaged in aberrant behavior due to unfulfilled desires of the heart and soul, how do we get off of that track and back on to a path of wholeness and prosperous living?

Well, Ms. Dunn provides a humorous yet sobering expose of her own trials with thoughtful insights that carry us into her journey in and lead us to her exit out of dysfunctional behavior born of unfulfilled expectations. Her prophetic insight will encourage and yet challenge you to gain your freedom from an eating disorder or any other malady whose root stems from our propensity to seek the approval of others, as we try to find our place of acceptance in the world. At the end of the day, she reminds us that there are two primary relationships that override all others: Love God with all your heart soul, and strength, and learn to love yourself. Without these relationships in order it is impossible to obey the command of Jesus to love others as you love yourself.

*Foreword*

This is truly a book of deliverance. Whether you are in the Lord or out of relationship with Him, you will be challenged to look at yourself and your relationship with God a little closer. A most interesting observation for me was how we can grow up "in church" and reach adolescence, adulthood, middle age, and old age without addressing some of these fundamental issues of brokenness. Could we have an eating disorder as "the Church"? Do we engage in "emotional eating" of the Word of the Lord and, therefore, never get satisfied? Well, you decide for yourself, as you read a cutting edge expose of a "son of God," who is determined to get it right, even at the expense of self-exposure. I believe you will find a measure of healing in this story; it's an axe with a sharp edge.

*Apostle Eric L. Warren*

Ambassador Ministries

Columbus, Ohio

# Little by Little, Bit by Bit

*For precept must be upon precept, precept upon precept; line upon line, line upon line; here a little, and there a little.*

Isaiah 28:10

Little by little, bit by bit,
Keep pressing toward the mark for the prize,
But don't you quit.
Keep on keeping on…
You'll make it through the storm
Little by little, bit by bit.

When you find that big old mountain right ahead of you,
And you just can't seem to get over or around it, no matter what you do;
You don't seem to have the faith to say, "Mountain, get out of my way!"
And you're so overwhelmed at times that you can't even pray,
Be like David and encourage yourself in the Lord and say,

## Fill My Heart

Little by little, bit by bit,
Keep pressing toward the mark for the prize,
But don't you quit.
Keep on keeping on…
You'll make it through the storm
Little by little, bit by bit.

You started your journey with the Lord and just wanted to bless,
But seems like life took a turn and is now one big mess.
Though things may not turn out the way you think they should,
Someday you'll look back and see that all things worked together for your good.
Just remember that no matter what happens that the Lord is good.

Little by little, bit by bit,
Keep pressing toward the mark for the prize,
But don't you quit.
Keep on keeping on…
You'll make it through the storm
Little by little, bit by bit.

Be encouraged and know the Lord will strengthen those who wait
Times may be hard, but you'll reap someday if you just don't faint.
Weeping may endure for night, but joy will surely come in the morning light
And remember these words: "Be strong in the Lord and power of his might."
You're more than a conqueror, so keep the faith and fight the good fight.

Little by little, bit by bit,
Keep pressing toward the mark for the prize,
But don't you quit.
Keep on keeping on…
You'll make it through the storm
Little by little, bit by bit.

*Little by Little, Bit by Bit*

Little by little, bit by bit,
Keep pressing toward the mark for the prize,
Little by little, bit by bit. Little by little, bit by bit. Little by little, bit by bit.

*Lonnell Johnson*

Used by Permission

# Table of Contents

Preface: Leaving Home .................................................................. 17

Chapter 1 ........................................................................................ 23
Here's the Skinny on Emotional Eating

Chapter 2 ........................................................................................ 27
This Thing Was Always Bigger Than Me

Chapter 3 ........................................................................................ 33
Come Unto Me and Rest

Chapter 4 ........................................................................................ 37
Why'd You Go and Do It, Eve?

Chapter 5 ........................................................................................ 43
The Fat Belongs To God: Sacrificing What I "Deserve" for What He Desires

Chapter 6 ........................................................................................ 49
Desperate Truths

Chapter 7 ........................................................................................ 57
Kill the Fatted Calf

Chapter 8 ........................................................................................ 63
Naked and Ashamed

Chapter 9 ........................................................................................ 69
Tried In the Balance…and Found "Wanting"

Chapter 10 ...................................................................................... 75
I Came For Form — And If I Can Manage It — Fashion

Chapter 11 ...................................................................................... 79
Hide Me: Developing the Lifestyle of Weightless Worship.

Chapter 12 ...................................................................................... 87
Sweeter Than Honey — Prayers to Pray Along the Way

# *Preface: Leaving Home*

I never even realized that I was fat until I left home. Seriously. Fat had, and continues to have far less to do with physical weight than it did with my perception of its significance. And in many ways, I did not begin to perceive its significance until I left home. What's more, fat had far more to do with the comparisons I made when I started to believe that weight distinguished me from others. Now, it occurs to me that "distinguished" may be far too polite a word for a book that I hope will help you to confront your own truths about weight. What I really mean to say is that in my case, fat meant different, and different meant inferior, or so it seemed when I left home.

I grew up in the South. We believed in sweet tea long before popular restaurants discovered its lure. And we have been known to fry the most unsuspecting of vegetables and smother still others in gravy. Sausage remains a staple in the breakfasts of many, but then what else would you expect to hold together a fresh baked biscuit? And how do I begin to describe the things that can be done to an otherwise harmless fruit once covered in butter and sugar and baked into a delectable pastry crust—cobbler. Early on, diet conditioned me to consider excess as acceptable and to ignore my growing problem—fat.

Now, I can already hear collective resistance. Why, you're wondering, would I refer to myself using such an oppressive term? I use it—and it has ceased to oppress me, by the way—precisely because it no longer holds the power it did when wielded by my enemy. I know this because I've tried others, all as uncomfortable and ill-fitting as Saul's armor on David. I've tried "overweight," "full-figured," "big-boned," "large," "plus-sized"—but none of them are as expressive, none as innocent nor as impotent as "fat." For one thing, fat has not always meant what it means in our current cultural context. In many cultures outside of America's, it still does not. I think we've developed the range of words we use to describe weight partly because of that. Consider too that gradual increases in the average size of American women have revolutionized the fashion industry. While it's still the case that fashion trends are driven by styles designed for small bodies, bigger ones have made an undeniable impact and constitute a significant portion of the market.

All said, we simply don't recognize our differences until we leave home. Beyond recognizing them, though, we have to be taught that they are, in one way or another, objectionable before we assign a negative value to them. We are only condemned by differences we are conscious of. Once we become conscious of difference, especially of our alleged inferiority because of it, that awareness tends to make us self-conscious. I spent three months in Nigeria several years ago, and it profoundly altered my experience and understanding of beauty. I saw women of every shade of "black" imaginable—all beautiful. And while I did not converse with most of them, everything in their carriage and composure makes me believe that they'd not internalized the consciousness of complexion that my American sisters have. Even more affirming, they were every shape and size—all beautiful. And so, I dared to bare my arms in Nigeria! In some very real ways, I found myself back at home at last.

You see, family creates the cultural context for acceptance. As one of the earliest and most enduring reflections of corporate identity—our families define us. And when we leave home, particularly under less than ideal circumstances, we sometimes struggle to redefine ourselves. And so, in lots of ways, *Fill My Heart* is about leaving home, not just literally, but emotionally. Part reflection on Biblical stories involving food, part the story of myself, it represents a radical departure from comfort. I challenged myself, as I hope this book will challenge you, to examine the ways in which the comforts of home may have now become uncomfortably weighty limits in your life.

When I began to write this book, I presumed it would lead me rather quickly along a journey toward my ideal weight. In fact, I began writing it with every intention of holding the book signing just after my first marathon or rock climbing adventure or salsa dance class. I imagined its publication following any number of things that I'd convinced myself would only happen, or could only happen, after I'd lost a considerable amount of weight. But since God so often has unusual things in mind for us—things we might never conceive of ourselves—He surprised me.

The writing of this book has marked one of the most difficult journies of my entire life. Whether with conventional or so called "crash" diets, I found myself losing weight time after time but never with lasting results. Even my occasional successes were undermined by a lack of persistence that defied reason. More times than I can or care to recount, I came close to success, losing 20-30 pounds and practicing new patterns for a few months. Invariably, though, I experienced what I now recognize as self-sabotage. Perhaps I returned to the familiar because it was—well—familiar.

Familiar things have an almost irresistibly comforting pull on us. They sing the comforting lullabies of home to us, transporting us to places where we hardly need our words or senses at all, a supreme irony, since so much of what appeals to us about food is just that—descriptive and sensual. We find ourselves falling in love with it—the way it looks or smells or feels—and all of that is without even beginning to account for its emotional impact. And if it weren't for the exotic names of some dishes, I'm certain we would never consume them! We fall in love with food, not because of what it is, but because of what it represents. Writing this book,

I discovered a similar truth. It was not only that I had to lose the physical weight, but that I redefine the emotional and sensual traps, the ways of feeling about food that had held my weight in place. I had to begin to understand what food represented before I could begin to manage what it would "be" to me.

I have since concluded that I will be losing weight for some time to come; at very least, I will have to be intentional about diet and exercise for the rest of my life. But it was the writing of this book that helped me discover the relationships between weight gain and the emotions behind it. My prayer is that you will, likewise, feel your way to fullness—spirit, soul and body.

As you read this book, you will no doubt discover the unhealthy ties you've built between food, and if not food, anything else that has weighed you down. I suspect you'll want to look at your own family food history to determine how early behaviors and patterns got their start. Like the families we're born into, attitudes toward food and any consequent issues with weight are inherited. But in Christ, we're never simply stuck with whatever we've been handed. We can always exchange what we no longer need for the more excellent. I encourage you to take the time to savor the questions at the end of each chapter. They will honestly provoke you to rethink the chapter you've just read. In this case, they should help you to reevaluate your own and your family's ties to food as you purposefully create new ones that free you to be your best self!

## *Food for Thought*

1. Describe your family in terms of body size and image. How much emphasis was placed on outward appearance and with what impact on the way you see yourself?

2. What did your family understand/express about body size/image? Were they essentially accepting? If not, how have their beliefs influenced your self image?

3. Are there activities you've postponed until you reach some goal? What do you expect to be different once you reach that goal? What could happen if you simply acted now?

# Here's the Skinny on Emotional Eating

We are all familiar with emotional eating. It's the sort that, rather than fueling the body, fills the heart. In short, it becomes the means by which *we feel* rather than *fuel*. When we're eating emotionally, food becomes the means of addressing or expressing unmnet emotional needs. We naturally gravitate toward certain "comfort" foods because they remind us of familiar times or places or even people. The trouble is, sometimes those times, places and people are more fantastic than familiar. Who has not smelled freshly baked bread and been instantly reminded of her mother's kitchen, or inhaled the aroma of grilling meat and not been miraculously returned to his childhood BBQs? Are those emotional memories "real" in the sense that they take us back to actual kitchens or backyards? Sometimes they are. But it's just as likely that those familiar smells act as triggers of what we wish had been.

Let's face it, the original intention of food was that it would fuel our bodies and permit us to fulfill our earthly mandates. But like any counterfeit, emotional eating promises what it can never deliver—fullness. The smell of that bread baking or of that delicious steak grilling takes us back, not so much to what was, but to what we wish to recreate in the present. Oh, it's not that our mothers never baked or that our families never gathered around a grill anxiously awaiting the first bite of summer. And I don't mean to suggest that all our positive, sensual experiences of food are imagined or illicit. I simply want to begin with this understanding: eating is essentially a physical necessity. If we expect it to feed something else—whether spirit or soul—we will never be full.

Only in writing this book did it occur to me that man's entire existence is bound up with this truth. We were created of three parts: spirit, soul, and body. In that order, they were meant to predominate, to permit us to establish and maintain the dominion of God in the earth. We were to dress, keep, subdue, and rule the earth, to be fruitful and, finally, multiply. The single restriction in this idyllic environment was that we not eat from the tree of the knowledge of good and evil. That's because it was not simply physical, though it clearly bore physical fruit. After all, it could be seen and shared! It was physical. But it was far more than that.

However else she was deceived, Eve got one thing right. The Bible says that she understood that the tree was "good for food," that it was "pleasant to the eyes," and that it was "to be desired to make one wise" (Genesis 3:6). In other words, *this* tree appealed not only to the body, but to the soul and spirit as well. This was clearly no mere mid-afternoon snack! But when God intends us to nourish our bodies, he doesn't want us doing so with things that inflate our egos or create a false sense of spiritual security. I believe that's why he uses food so often throughout the Bible to deal with motives of the heart. It is not to be used to isolate the poor from the wealthy but is to be made equally available to whoever will "come and dine" at his invitation. It is not meant to hold us hostage to our greater needs, the ones that would compel us to join a multitude and follow past exhaustion and hunger. Rather, it is meant to revive us so that our following is of desire and not desperation. And it is certainly not meant to invade our feasts and most sacred celebrations as a means of satisfying the appetite. It is simply and yet profoundly significant of the intangible, living bread—the very presence of God.

*Here's the Skinny on Emotional Eating*

The trouble with food for emotional eaters is that "it is good for (far more than) food." It begins to fill needs of the soul, and sometimes the spirit, contrary to its created purpose. God is serious about consumption—always has been. He relates outcomes to intake. Here's a good example of how He does that: He often sets a vision of tremendous success before us—a veritable "Eden" of whatever abundance he wants us to rule over—only to develop our character by mediating our intake—spiritual, emotional or physical—until we model not only His outcome but His intention. He places us in the midst of abundance, but then urges restraint so that we are "in and not of" our surroundings. Ultimately, He wants us not to be mastered by our appetites but to master them.

This is exactly how He developed the character of many of those who've taught us crucial life lessons. For Abraham, the matter was not so much that he produce a son or even a nation, but that he would become a model of faith in the face of otherwise insurmountable odds. And with Moses, it wasn't just that he deliver Israel from Egypt, but that he would become a model of persistence in the face of denial. And who can forget Joseph and his dreams? The issue was not so much that he rise in leadership and authority over his brothers, but that he perfect the profession of truth—even when his dreams seemed to escape him.

If we are ever to master emotional eating, it will be similarly. How do you handle having had a promise made to you, a promise that is then deferred for years? Do you insist upon gratifying your own needs or do you continue to refocus your needs in response to the original vision God has set? And how do you handle being told no outright? Do you simply resolve that the thing can't be done—that you can never be free? Do you manage betrayal by becoming bitter, or do you determine to let it make you better? Those are all essential questions in how you will permit God to shape your character and your body. He often wants to do both at once.

Writing this book, I realized that physical weight loss would not be its cause or consequence. Losing the weight would not legitimize my story more or less, and the writing could not possibly produce a truth that miraculously caused weight to drop off. I did, however, find an arresting connection between the two. Writing created and continues to create a context for self-discovery, for discovering what has been hidden. And so, as I write, I am uncovering myself—literally. The weight loss could not have preceded the uncovering. That would have made the discovery a right to earn, a privilege reserved for the physically "perfect." And the weight loss could not wait for the completion of the book—as if the book were some sort of prescriptive "how to" manual. Instead, the two are growing to be one. At times, the discoveries contribute to changes in my diet and exercise. At other times, I'm sure that the changes in my body will lead to further discoveries—some pleasant, some painful. Either way, I will write, even as I have for the past year. The result is not simply *Fill My Heart*—but a heart that continues to grow more full every day. May your heart experience the same fullness as you read the remaining pages.

## Food for Thought

1. If you are an emotional eater, what emotions are you avoiding and why? What makes it difficult or "unacceptable" to express the actual emotions?

2. Do you identify with any of the Biblical characters mentioned in this chapter—Abraham, Moses, or Joseph? If so, in what similar ways have you been tested?

# 2

# This Thing Was Always Bigger Than Me

I cannot remember a time when I have not struggled with my weight, a time when I was not painfully conscious of not measuring up because of it. I have equally few memories of proudly or guiltlessly celebrating my body, delighting in its unique curves and slopes. I have mostly wished that it were not so, or at least that it was not so much.

It began, they tell me, at my birth. "Mrs. Dunn," the nurses joked, "You're going to have to buy a cow!" Apparently, they'd never encountered an infant who demanded more than the three-ounce ration of milk and insistently at that. I did. And I was loud about it. I cried until they fed me, and fed me, and fed me. It never once occurred to them that I wasn't hungry—at least not for milk.

Even then, what I was thirsty for wasn't physical but, I am convinced, spiritual. In fact, I am convinced more than ever that every heart hunger is really a hunger for Christ. Why else the mindless pursuit of that which often does not satisfy? Power? Money? Sex? Or why the endless lust for something, anything that promises to fill the void of the heart only to wound it again? What makes us return to the same "plate" or "pitcher," or whatever the culture's current menu offering happens to be, time after time, even when the last "meal" clearly left us empty and broken? The greatest irony and our greatest deception is that we continue to think that we're full. We have, as an Old Testament prophet declares, mistaken "broken cisterns for the fountain of life," when we might have been truly full had we only gone to the living well.

We have to feed whatever the actual appetite is with whatever we're actually hungry for. Otherwise, emptiness only continues to masquerade as fullness, lulling us into complacency. We seem so full, so satisfied, if only by that which we never even wanted. As an infant, I must have eventually gotten what I wanted in the way of milk, probably long before those well-intentioned nurses stopped feeding me. And full of what I hadn't wanted to begin with, I must have eventually quieted down and brought less attention to myself. I imagine that my quiet compliance with their expectations brought even more gratuitous gifts of milk! And so, very early it seems, I was learning to quiet down and drink deeply from the "broken cistern" of emotional eating. It led to a lifetime of putting food in an inappropriate place—my heart. And with so much food displacing so many emotions, I became as quiet as one possibly could.

Ironically, growing up in a noisy church, a traditional Holiness one, made that fairly easy. There was the obvious, now anachronistic, emphasis on what women wore and the far more lasting impression made by the teaching to "wear the world as a loose garment." And so, clothing fascinated me early on. So much of my early religious education concerned the differences in what men and women could and could not wear, that clothing gradually became a vehicle for my ongoing monologue of resistance. Oh, I was quiet, but that did not mean that I was genuinely compliant! While I conceded outwardly to church expectations, as a teen, I became less and less personally engaged in my faith. External conformity. Internal confusion. While it began as a matter of clothing, "covering up" became an emotional coping strategy. Suppressing the questions I should have asked but could never find the voice for, I retreated further into religion and rote behavior. Neither brought me any real satisfaction, though I pretended well. Of necessity, my earliest ways of understanding God were abstract. They centered on how vast the world was, and how vast God must be to love all of it, but only in an implicit and impersonal way did I understand the love of God. My experience of God was like the worst of junk food diets; you can eat and eat, but never become full. In fact, the more you eat, the hungrier you seem to become. I wanted to know and understand God, but my religious "diet" simply left me malnourished.

And who could survive the hallways of a junior high school without a clear and definite sense of the love of God? No one! Junior high brought with it a very personal need for God. Had I understood then what I am coming to understand now, I might have invited Him to sit with me at the smart kids' lunch table and protect me from the daily tirades of the "bad kids" who knew my parents were preachers, making it highly unlikely that I would curse back at them or swing when swung at. But the notion that God could be as close as the next locker was a foreign one to me. My thinking went something like this: God is love, or at least He loves the world. But if that's really the case, why the excruciating pain of public showers after gym or modern dance assignments that would remain the bane of my existence in PE or the rope? How could a truly loving God permit the rope? ☺ My experience of love or what I presumed to represent love was dramatically different from my understanding of it. In my understanding, I wanted to believe that God loved me no matter what my size or level of physical ability. But junior high led me to believe otherwise, and tipping the scales at just under 200 pounds by then, I somehow doubted.

From a distance of some years, I can clearly see the flaws in my logic—negative thinking patterns planted, no doubt, by an enemy who never meant to see this book come to fruition. What I somehow learned by the grace of God is that His love cannot be simply reduced to the good fortune or favor of men, or in this case, adolescent boys. We are not more loved of God when we are more accepted or praised of men. In fact, the opposite is far more often true.

From an emotional distance, I can also see that adolescence was simply the time for those plaguing experiences, that all or most of us shared a common but silent self-loathing. But what can now be seen as "common" from the perspective of the adult was cloudy from the perspective of the teenaged girl. My discomfort in my own body resulted in a discomfort with God (whom I must have expected to miraculously rush in at 5th period and save me from PE!) As a result, there proceeded other serious doubts about all that was right—or not—in His world. I was especially doubtful about the parts of it that seemed out of balance, unkempt, unkept. It must have been about the same time that food began to respond very personally to my insistent questions about how things got to be that way.

In junior high, food was definitely love. Food was an unfailing and absolutely faithful comforter. It hid me. It was omnipresent and all-powerful. Food was "god." And thus, my faith in food was conceived. It was not nearly so lockstep, but if you understand the role that food played in comforting and confirming this small (inside, at least) girl who hadn't yet found her voice, though she was always talking, and who hadn't quite found her "flow" though she must have always been moving, then you understand why for years, I found "god" in food.

I can remember older church women sometimes saying the simple words "we see you" which was to say, go somewhere and sit down, make yourself less conspicuous, less noisy—less. And so inwardly, I did. My own voice grew more and more quiet, and the seemingly irresistible call of food grew louder and louder. And in the increasing quiet—some of it social conditioning, some of it my nature—I became an interior sort, conversing mostly with myself. It does not surprise me now that this tendency toward the sedentary coupled with the constant business of church and a family business created what then seemed like a "natural" bent toward introspection rather than activity.

And only now do I better understand those church women's attempts to quiet me. They meant only to educate me to the "facts" of my existence early so that I might have an easier time being.

## This Thing Was Always Bigger Than Me

Growing up in a Holiness church demanded no less. We were an amalgam of antitheses—all at once we were less and more. We ran things, but were never expected to take the credit for doing so. And while our voices were loud in the choir stand and, occasionally, even the pulpit, they were all but silent when it came to church administration. But even outside of church, the women I knew were consumed with church work. They were, after all, giving themselves sacrificially to the up-building of the kingdom. I imagine all of that up-building cultivated quite an appetite, since a great number of them, as I recall, were fat. All of that church work brought with it a busy-ness that sometimes denied them the opportunity to simply be women. There were Sunday School teachings to prepare, and convention guests to host, and an endless array of literary program details to attend to. And then there were hats to match to purses, choirs to lead, and money trees to make! And none of that diminished the other sorts of work I saw them accomplish. My own mother owned a business, a flower shop she founded and managed and loved. Between the church work and the other work, not to mention the care and feeding of a family, I don't know when she had time to be, much less be more—unless it was in church. There, she was an icon. Virtually every church woman I knew was. They were literally larger than life. I admired them, but secretly, I wanted to be less. Less busy, less otherworldly—just less.

Now here's the thing—there's truth in understanding that God intends for us to become less of ourselves. As He increases, we decrease in so many ways. But less *of* ourselves is not less *than* ourselves. What I saw and what I'm sure contributed to much emotional eating early on was frustrated vision. In the absence of real influence or assignment, much of the church activity I observed seemed simply to be busy work. It was useful, for sure, but mostly to those who received the benefits of it—not to those who completed it. Activity is supposed to bring us fulfillment, not simply because it's personally gratifying, but because it locks us into kingdom purpose. It is supposed to make us more than ourselves—more corporately than we could ever have been individually.

Nothing creates a bigger space in the heart than mindless activity. If we are not doing what we were created to do, we will fill the vacuum of purpose with food. If we are not acknowledging what we really need, we will fill the absence with junk—literally and spiritually. If we are ever to conquer emotional eating—and we are—we have to begin by identifying what we're really hungry for. The abundant life we're promised in Christ means becoming less of the selves we've been reduced to by rote, religious thinking and becoming more of the beautiful creation God originally intended. More is exactly what God created us for! We are created in His image and if He has the capacity to become more, then so do we! In myriad ways, we reflect His glory by becoming more and more and more—not less. May you become more, starting today!

## Food for Thought

1. How have early (mis)understandings about God influenced your relationship with food?

2. If not food, what else have you used as a substitute for relationship with God?

3. What is the "more" that God created you for? Have you been secretly hoping to become less when what He's really calling for is more? If so, what gets in your way?

# Come Unto Me and Rest

God's intention for us has always been that we be more. But somehow, like Eve, we twist perfectly positive truths into very damaging lies. And if we swallow one, thinking we're consuming the other, we can end up with an awful case of spiritual indigestion. Consider, for instance, how comfortable most of us have become with our busy-ness. We've thoroughly digested the lie that more is actually more—more meetings, more tasks, more objectives— more fruitful? Not always. We've all but lost the art of genuinely quieting ourselves, not just shutting ourselves up or suppressing ourselves, and it's costly.

There is a direct correlation between our rush toward—well, whatever it is that we're rushing toward—and our inability to get quiet inside. The hurrying about often keeps us from slowing down long enough to genuinely feel hunger pangs—not for food, but for whatever it is we'd really like to be filled with. I still believe that it's God, and that more than anything, we really want to be filled with Him. But if we never learn to distinguish between feelings of physical hunger and feelings of spiritual or emotional hunger, we may never be satisfied.

I am unquestionably an emotional eater. When I began this book, and even through earlier periods of attentiveness to diet or exercise, I made an uncomfortable discovery. I very seldom felt hunger. More often than not, I ate without any regard to what my body actually needed, but with rather acute attention to what my emotions wanted. And even they were prohibited from a wide range of healthy expressions. I ate, not so much in response to emotional highs and lows, but to prevent them. The fuller I was physically, the less I felt emotionally. Was I ever empty!

There's good reason to believe that the great majority of Americans are living equally empty lives. One has to make a conscientious effort to avoid the increased media coverage of what has been called a national crisis of obesity, its impact on health, projections for the next generations, and so on. With more than half of us overweight or obese, we are clearly a culture eating its way to emptiness. More recently still, we hear that there are connections between weight gain and poor sleep patterns. Small wonder—God created us for balance. Rest is meant to permit the body to sort out its various impulses; it's an intentional and necessary break from activity that gives the systems an opportunity to know what they've expended and to what extent they need to be restored. But if we are neither eating nor sleeping adequately, we can easily lose that balance.

And it seems little better for those of us who say we hunger and thirst after God. A good, hard look around our churches will confirm that we're as affected by misaligned relationships with food or improper exercise and rest as everyone else, perhaps more so. For much of the church, a dangerous escapist mentality has persisted, masquerading as spiritual zeal. Aside from its theological implications, it has fostered a fairly consistent disregard for many things earthly, most especially the physical body. The rationale goes something like this: If we are going to shed it at our great "exodus" anyway, why be so concerned for it? But that is the biggest lie ever told!

We must begin to tell the truth. We have, again, forsaken the fountains of living water and have crowded around broken cisterns. In our restlessness, we have wandered aimlessly from one stagnant pool to the next so that now we are not simply thirsty, but weary as well. *Fill My Heart*, then, is more than a book on weight loss—it is an urgent, prophetic call to return to cool streams and places of genuine rest. What would it be like, for instance, to begin to create an atmosphere for eating similar to the one we create for worship? What would it look like, in other words, to take eating as seriously as God obviously does? What might happen if, instead of rushing through the drive-through, or hurriedly consuming dinner from a microwave container, we actually sat down? Wouldn't we have to focus on the experience, and might we not be fuller because of it? And what's making us rush so anyway? I realize that multiple responsibilities can occasionally obligate our time more than we'd like them to, but if we are never resting and consciously focusing on what we are consuming, we will probably never be full. I recall more than a few days when, in the bustle of one activity after another, I have actually forgotten to eat. But I can recall a greater number of days when, similarly, I have forgotten what I've already consumed. It's clear that I ate something, but I was so unconscious of it that whatever it was, it had little impact.

As I experience remarkable changes in my mind and body, I am finally connecting two unforgettable biblical truths about rest and eating. It has always amazed me that when He was about his Father's business, Jesus actually removed himself from the rush and spent significantly less time in the busy-ness we sometimes use to define our spirituality. And it has never ceased to amaze me that when He sat down to "break bread," it was no haphazard effort. Dining meant drawing away, reclining even, for long periods of time. Aside from times of complete fasting, there is nothing that suggests that Jesus saw the restorative times He spent dining and reclining with His disciples as any less significant than when He was teaching or healing or delivering people. In fact, the table often served as His de facto "pulpit" and the appetite as His text. We would do well to take the consumption of literal bread as seriously as we do receiving His living word.

And so, while this is clearly a book about weight loss, it is also a book about becoming our best, most rested selves in Christ. As I write, and as you read, may we learn to rest long enough to identify the real sources of hunger in our lives and to only fill them with what truly satisfies.

## *Food for Thought*

1. When was the last time you really rested—just stopped, sat still—even for a few minutes? Try it now, and journal whatever God speaks to you about food.

2. How much time do you spend on meals? From selection, to preparation, to consumption—do you find yourself rushing or slowing down to savor the experience of eating?

3. Are you sleeping well? If not, what might be making you restless? Does your night-time restlessness have an impact on your day-time eating habits?

# Why'd You Go and Do It, Eve?

Of all the ways God might have chronicled the departure and descent of the human race, He centered the story on our rebellion, and He recounted our rebellion as a commentary on consumption. For many, that will seem theologically incorrect, like some simplistic reduction of a biblical doctrine that scholars and saints have haggled over for hundreds of years. But for those of us who have struggled or still struggle with the temptation to eat what we should not, there is an intimate understanding of rebellion that can never be separated from what we consume.

That's because there is an internal mechanism for most of us that indicates when we're off course. At some level, we know that the second serving—and the third—are wrong, but they are just so appealing. The question is—to what? What is the temptation to overeat appealing to? Perhaps a look back at Genesis will give us some useful insights.

We're familiar with the story. God created everything with intention, including the garden in which he placed Adam and Eve to rule. In that garden, He planted every imaginable sort of tree, but forbade them to eat of just one of them—the one in the midst of the garden. Here, I think even placement is significant. Matters of appetite are central—they cannot be avoided and out from them radiate an enormous number of choices, once we have mastered the one that is most central. In the rush to discern the significance of the tree of the knowledge of good and evil, many of us have failed to see the significance of what preceded God's forbidding Adam to eat from it. It was freedom. Of every other tree, He explained, they had the liberty to eat freely (Genesis 2:16). The single restriction was explicit and exclusive. There must have been hundreds, perhaps thousands of trees from which they could have eaten—but they desired this one. That illicit desire was ignited in no small part by the serpent's subtlety, just as there are countless food advertisements to contend with, not to mention an entire culture of license and licentiousness best (though not exclusively) expressed through the "all you can eat" phenomenon. But ultimately, the choice was theirs.

I still remember my first "all you can eat" buffet. I was met at the door by a veritable smorgasbord of sights and smells—talk about sensual overload! Truth, or rather, deception is—it wasn't even particularly good food as I think of it now. It was no one's "specialty," no chef's daily delight. There was just a seemingly endless supply and no restriction on how much of it one could consume. This particular one was famous for its fried chicken. While a public sense of self-consciousness prevented me from literally eating all I could, my cousins seemed undaunted. Perhaps because they were male, and not particularly overweight—they ate, and ate, and ate. Not terribly unusual for teenaged boys, I know, but still reflective of how we'll often behave differently than we typically would once restraints are removed.

At some point, "all you can eat" became "all you care to eat," a subtle but significant difference. "Can" is a matter of ability. "Care to" makes it a matter of will and emotion. Again, there is usually an internal mechanism that indicates when we're eating more than we should. And at some base level, the elemental offensiveness of "all you can eat," that is to say, all one has the capacity to pack in, must have given way to the more socially and psychologically acceptable "all you care to eat." This phrase, intentionally or not, expressed an underlying spiritual truth, one God hoped Adam and Eve would learn in the garden of Eden: eating is integrally expressive of the will. Consumers are now making a choice—having things our way. And that's precisely what Eve's rebellion against God signified—the age-old desire to have our own way.

But it represented even more. She not only twisted God's words, she added to them making them more restrictive than He ever intended them to be. And when her deception is revealed, she feels justified in blaming everyone but herself. In the face of lives that sometimes go in directions we never anticipated or simply refuse to go where we'd will them to, we become rebellious and angry and frustrated. But when we're angry and frustrated, or even when we're hurting, it's not good enough just to rebel. Most often, we begin to lie to ourselves. Did God really say...? Or, surely He could not have meant.... And if deceiving ourselves is not bad enough, we begin to lie to others.

One of the most profound lessons I learned from a famous weight loss program was simply this: accountability counts. When I was required to record everything I consumed, I lied more than any good Christian would care to admit! And it wasn't just that I left things out of my weekly journal. That was fairly common. While I make no excuse for that, I am much more troubled by my even more subtle deceptions. More often than not, before I became serious about my weight loss, I would record what I'd consumed, but I'd conveniently neglect to record portions. Or I would tell most of the real truth, but add my own as well. Surely a couple of glasses of water must be as good as eight, I'd convince myself. And a few vegetables—well, I could always double up on the carrots tomorrow, right?

Eve acted in exactly this way—subtly. Not only was she not to eat of the tree, she explained to the serpent, she was not even supposed to touch it. You see, rebellion always has a way of exacting something from the rebel and from the authority figure. Rationalization indefinitely postpones genuine confrontation. Even as she conversed with the serpent, Eve was well on the way, not only toward entangling Adam, but also toward denying her responsibility once God confronted her. And God, who I'm convinced would have been willing to forgive had there only been repentance, was compelled instead to punish.

But rationalization only *postpones* the confrontation. And so, when it inevitably comes, whether with God, the great balancer, or even with a lesser scale, it almost invariably comes to break us of a rebellious or inordinate desire for power. I've by no means meant to suggest that original sin plunged the entire race into separation from God simply over food. But then and now, food represents power. "You shall be like gods," the serpent whispered. "Your eyes shall be opened and you'll become wise," he seduced. To Eve, and often to us, eating represents access to power. The question is, what sort? What power does consumption produce? Beyond fueling the body and enabling it to function, what sort of power do we get from eating?

We know this much—the satisfaction of feeling full literally lulls the body, tells it that all is well. Eating sets off the chemical chain of events that communicate to our brain that we are not starving. But what sort of power does overeating produce? Past the chemical reactions, what does the feeling of over fullness communicate?

Quite often, I found it to produce numbness. I found food to numb emotions I would rather not have felt at the time and to squelch confrontations I would rather have avoided altogether. If fullness creates for the body the sense that all is well, somehow, over fullness created the sense that all would be well in the future. It had the capacity, in my experience at least, to reach over into uncertainty and doubt, and often into outright lack to convince me, nevertheless, that all would be well. Say what you will, food has prophetic implications.

I'm sure that this is what Israel experienced in the wilderness when God was providing manna for them. They desired onions and leeks, the food of their past, or quail, suggestive of the richer diet they anticipated in the "promised" land. But I am struck most by their attempts to convert what was meant to be daily bread into something entirely different—to pervert and extend its use past the day on which it was given. If you're familiar with what happened when Israel collected more than a single day's manna, you cannot deny that food has prophetic implications. The manna they collected in excess spoiled and produced maggots. Excess produces corruption. We have only to look honestly at the myriad of health problems caused by our national crisis of obesity—hypertension, diabetes, etc.—to confirm this.

The first challenge of the character and integrity of Jesus Christ was to eat what he should not. Satan hoped Jesus would experience corruption were He to consent to making stones into bread in His own wilderness. Likewise, in some way or other, every temptation is a test of the appetite. In this case, bread was no more significant than the specific sort of tree Eve ate from. The issue was and always will be access to power. And in response to the temptation to eat what he should not, Christ replies with a more excellent kind of nourishment—living bread, or the bread of presence.

The significance of this passage in terms of a right relationship with food is this: only fullness with the Word and presence of God will withstand the temptation to fullness of *any* other sort. Both spiritual and physical fullness, not to mention hunger, require that we remain in our present with God. Going past it typically means that we have failed or refused to trust that when we really need it, more will be available. I'm more convinced than ever of the absolute necessity of the phrase from what is commonly called "The Lord's Prayer." "Give us this day our daily bread" means precisely that: be fully present today, God. And in the ways that I can never fully anticipate, be fully present again tomorrow. And that is exactly what God has promised to be.

## *Food for Thought*

1. What are the sources of any rebellion you've demonstrated in your relationship with God or others?
2. Think about a time when you knew you were beyond the boundaries—intentionally or not—in your eating. What

pushed you "there" and what was the rationale, the story you told yourself, as you went "there"?

# The Fat Belongs To God: Sacrificing What I "Deserve" for What He Desires

There are a great many things we'll do for love that we will not do for any other cause—and sacrifice is one of them. As a child, I was often perplexed by the story of Cain and Abel. Perpetually identifying and identified with the underdog, I just wanted Cain to be able to win! Why, I mused, if he'd brought from the crop he'd produced, couldn't his offering be acceptable? Did God simply prefer flocks to fruits? Worse yet, did He play favorites? Was there something about Abel He just liked more than Cain? I wrestled with this thought for some time.

Well, I've since learned much about love and sacrifice—and at least a little more about offerings. And while the Old Testament is full of interesting directives, and even more full of meaning, I'm sure, for the historically and culturally intelligent reader, the single most recurring theme I've found is that God expects what is first and what is fat.

From oldest times, there have been restrictions of one sort or another on what we consume versus what we sacrifice. I will certainly not attempt an explication of Old Testament offerings, or of injunctions against one food or the other, as I am no expert in those matters. I will, however, speak of the inspiration I derived and often did even as a child from what worship teaches me about eating and about giving.

I still have my first Bible. I think it was a birthday gift, but whenever I received it, I fell in love with it. It was an illustrated translation, a paraphrase of the Living Bible and easy to read. I was most enamored of the front-cover picture of Jesus carrying a lamb. This Bible became my first adventure book! You might think a girl of ten or so would seek out Psalms or bright New Testament passages to memorize, but those have never been my strength. I loved Leviticus! I know—it seems odd now—but something about routines intrigues me to this day. The meticulous preparation of offerings, the exactness in application of sacrifices, the almost militaristic order in all things temple-driven—that's the stuff of drama—and the stuff I loved to mull over as a child learning about God. In some way or other, food has always been relative to order—or disorder—in my life. Whether or not this was what fascinated me about Leviticus, I can't say. But it's clear that the way God spoke of fat was, well, nothing short of awe-inspiring.

Fat was elevated to the level of the sublime. It was reserved. To be reverenced—representative even—of the very best of the sacrifice. It was, in Old Testament terms, what kept the offering burning upon the altar and what, to my childlike imagination, made quite the dramatic show of flames as the priest laid it there. If, after all, fat was forbidden and could only be consumed by God—it must have been very special indeed. I confess, my most consonant moments were far from spiritual ones. Sacrificial Object Lesson #1? Dinner at Western Sizzler. How anticipation built as I placed my order, selected my beverage, choose the customary iceberg lettuce and carrot salad and, if permitted, chose a dessert. But consummation came when steak met grill! How fat sizzles! It causes flames to leap, fueling their elegant and captivating dance.

## The Fat Belongs To God

Now I should apologize right now to any Biblical scholars reading—not to mention any vegetarians—but right there in Western Sizzler, I had my first spiritual revelation! What Abel brought to God, "fat portions from some of the firstborn of his flocks," was what is to characterize every true gift and every sacrificial offering. God always wants what is first and what is fat.

Giving what comes first is complicated for most of us. We balk at handing over what we're somehow convinced will run out before we've received our adequate portion. Whether it's money or food or something else, we worry that there will never be enough. And if by some chance there is enough, we worry that what we most desire will have been consumed by that time. Giving what comes first requires the kind of trust that, for someone who struggles with food, can come with great difficulty. After all, one of the primal promptings to consume what we should not is the still, small voice that there will not be enough. And I don't just mean food.

I heard a message recently on famine that sparked some critical questions. How do I behave when I am hungry? And more importantly, how do I behave when I realize that there is little to no chance of my supplying my own need? Let's be honest, the ultimate test of faithfulness comes not in the time or place of plenty. There, we secretly—if erroneously—believe our own sufficiency to be enough. But even when we are not so foolish as this, the presence of plenty can still subconsciously lull us into the belief that our basic instincts will never really be tested. It's difficult to account for how we'll really behave in a time of lack when we have only experienced plenty. Perhaps that is one of the reasons why God permits us to experience famines—and again—not just of food.

Giving what comes first requires ultimate trust. Trust says "I won't attempt self-sufficiency before surrendering what remains to you." But that level of trust can be hard to come by when you've failed—or been failed. Cain and Abel had an intimate understanding of both. They hadn't inherited paradise. And while I may be taking interpretive liberties here, there's little to stop me from imagining their parents, Adam and Eve, digging about for an existence, not only blaming each other, but still blaming God for having been put out of the garden. It cannot be considered an excuse, particularly since Abel figured out the sort of offering that pleased God, but it serves as one explanation at least, that Cain had probably never seen an example of humility or of repentance. He had no frame of reference for simply deferring and beginning again. And so, when he might have brought an acceptable offering of what was first and what was fat, he would not. If giving what is first is ultimately a test of trust, giving what is fat is ultimately a test of the will.

It is not simply that Cain did not or could not—he would not give an acceptable offering. Every act of preserving the fat for ourselves is ultimately an act of will. Even more than giving what is first, giving what is fat brings us face to face with who we think we are. Oh, we may give what is first, monetarily or during a fast even, in tithes, because we believe it to be what God deserves. But giving what is fat, or which constitutes excess, brings us to the question of how to handle what we think is rightfully ours. How do we handle our "right" to food? Knowingly or not, this is the very question we're dancing around when we presume that overeating is not to be compared with any other excess. For years, the Christian church has largely ignored the matter of overeating, justifying it as an acceptable "excess" unlike drug or alcohol abuse, smoking, sex or any number of other "less sacred" cows. As a result, we have failed not only to kill the giants that threatened past generations, but we have unwittingly fostered a license in the present generation that, only now, seems to be being challenged. It was this way with Cain. What began with his parent's rebellion surrounding the consumption of food now extended to his own rebellion—and eventually murder—surrounding the willful refusal to release what belonged to God.

Giving what is first and giving what is fat begins with a single acknowledgement that everything belongs to God. His way of seeing and engaging His creation and His people is abundance. There is enough and more than enough of everything. What is fat, though, is even more than that. And now, to return to my Western Sizzler revelation! Fat is excess. Fat is, to an offering, what extends the life of it, what keeps the smoke rising from it, what makes for the fragrance that indicates that something delicious has been surrendered.

As I learn to release my hold on food, I am also learning to give with less reserve, learning as Abel understood implicitly, to trade in the currency God accepts and spends—abundance. I'm much more full for it!

## Food For Thought

1. If you've ever struggled with believing there is enough of whatever your greatest need seemed to be, why did you? What kept you from believing that God's abundance included what you needed?

2. If you've ever struggled with not getting it right the first time like Cain, what might you do to challenge the way you deal with failure the next time you experience it?

# *Desperate Truths*

The pretty girls, it seemed, had secrets they never told. Junior high school marked them for induction into a society I only understood vicariously. I was surrounded by them, and so I caught snatches of their insider conversations, strained to decipher the meanings of their hushed giggling from the back of the bus, and was occasionally privy to their too loud protestations—"You betta stop it, boy! I'ma tell!" Even those of us who were excluded recognized a telltale lack of conviction in their voices. "Telling" was the farthest thing from their minds, unless announcing to the rest of us the pursuit of their highly sought after "booties" with mock cries of disgust counted as "telling." In those days, boys were in the habit of running past girls and pinching them. Of course, this resulted in the really cute boys' being chased, having book bags swung at them, or, at very least being smacked on the head. But apparently it was worth it, because the pretty girls and the cute boys reenacted this scene day after day of junior high.

Adolescence--in many ways, it's the most significant season of life—not so much for the kinds of exchanges I just related, but for what they represented. In every culture, there are those who are insiders and those who are outsiders. It can become far more complex than that, but in elemental ways, social groups function in essentially the same ways. And we learn our places early on. There are those who will argue that the first few years of life teach us most of what we'll ever learn, mostly because we are so inquisitive as children. Others will say that the wisest years by far are the middle ones—when we have lived long enough to discover what really matters, but not so long as to lack appreciation for what we've learned. The seasoned lives of still others are a testimony to the possibilities of even later life. Past the fragrant bud and beauty of youth, theirs is the sweet, fragrantly ripe fruit of the autumn years—wisdom. But I will always believe that whether spent as insiders or outsiders, the adolescent years have the greatest impact on how we examine the life behind us and on how we will predict or project what comes ahead.

One thing is certain—adolescence offers most of us our first real opportunity at self-definition. Before then, we have mostly lived the lives we were handed; after then, even our most intimate strivings can be motivated by social measures or fears that we won't measure up in some way. We wonder if we shouldn't have already become more or accomplished a certain something by a certain time. Often, we're pursued by regrets because of what we have done. Adolescence, then, presents the rare gift of choice irresistibly wrapped in independence. And that gift has been secured tightly by, of all things, innocence. For those who fearlessly seize it, and shake it like the wonderful present that it is, choice can be incredibly empowering.

At adolescence, our independence motivates us to break away from parental norms, gradually testing and proving our own values until we know that they fit us like a perfectly selected gift. Along the way, we fail a great deal, but retain just enough of childhood innocence to sustain hope. We know that we'll find our way to maturity—eventually.

If there is a natural adolescence, during which the insiders define and defend their standing, and during which the outsiders— sometimes openly, sometimes defending their own secrets—either long for admission or violently reject it, there must also be a spiritual adolescence. I think we hear of one such spiritual adolescence in the account of the woman with the issue of blood.

Now you may be wondering what her seemingly incurable condition has to do with persistent issues of weight. If you look closely, you'll find in her story a woman who understood desperate measures all too well. Mark's account describes how she had spent all her resources seeing countless doctors, none of whom could cure her. Now, I don't know one person who has struggled with weight who cannot intimately identify with her desperation. It takes only seconds to make a mental list of the programs and diets and procedures that promise success in weight loss, but that somehow fail. And I've tried many of them. I've counted calories and fat grams, consumed prepackaged foods, scrupulously swallowed refrigerated drinks—all with that same desperation. But it was not until I shook the sense of powerlessness that so often comes with dieting that I saw any real success.

You see, the central concept of most short-lived diets is change from the outside. We are led to believe that by eliminating certain foods—some altogether, others for limited amounts of time—we can affect lasting change. The trouble is that diets that only address the element of food never address the relationship we have with that food. They never require us to tell all the truth—only the symptoms.

I can imagine this woman going from doctor to doctor sharing essentially the same list of symptoms. "Yes, it began this way…and not just that, but there's the trouble with…uhm hhm, but I suppose I should also mention that…." And then, there were the shameful things that altogether defied articulation. With each attempt to retell her symptoms, with each failed measure, she must have lost a bit more of herself, a little more of her confidence. Persistent "issues" of weight can have a way of doing that too, of creating a sense of captivity to and powerlessness against an issue for which there is only one real cure—truth.

Perhaps that's why, as I confront the causes of my weight, I increasingly identify with the woman with this issue. Relegated by physical difference to the world of the outsiders, she examines the life behind her—and presses forward. She makes a choice. And she does a most daring thing in pressing toward Jesus. She exposes herself though she's fully aware of the likelihood of detection. Desperate issues require desperate measures.

If you've spent any time at all in church, you've heard her story preached a million times. At the height of their messages, most preachers regale us with stories of her courage, her persistence, her miraculous healing. The particularly artful ones detail her social rejection in ways that make her stench almost tangible to the congregation. They show us blood stained garments and leave us straining to hear the hushed tones of suspicious whispers that preceded her every time she stepped into public view. They bring us eye-to-eye with her exhausted face, sweat pooling there as she pressed though the crowd, dodging the steps of the people above who never even saw her. But they focus mostly on the very typical sermonic end, a resolution to suffering, because it is just that, a typical sermonic end. Of course, what they say is literally true, but the way they most often craft it, this woman's story becomes the consummation of sermonic desire. More than anything, they want her healed! And while her healing is certainly a relief for us all, it doesn't begin to measure up to what comes of her truth telling.

Truth leads to the consummation of this woman's desire—wholeness. Don't get me wrong, I am as moved as any by her healing, since for very personal and now more public purposes, I've considered weight loss to represent the consummation of my own, equally desperate desire. I've imagined that healing would look like arriving at my ideal weight, never shopping for convenience but for preference, telling more of the truth than I do without fear of attracting negative attention—and in many ways it will. But even more than my fascination with her healing or my own, I am struck by her desperate desire for wholeness and her willingness to tell the truth to get to it. Here was a woman, much like myself, who had everything and nothing to lose. In the course of her spiritual adolescence, she'd discovered that only the pretty girls could afford to keep their secrets. Desperate women must tell the truth!

In natural adolescence, we establish the ways we will choose to interpret whatever else happens to us from that point forward. Then and there we decide how we will see truth, often for the rest of our adult lives. We want to rid ourselves of pimples, or find just the right prom dress, to select and be selected by the most popular friends. In adolescence, these things typically reflect an end of our "issues." But, in spiritual adolescence, only truth telling moves us past healing to wholeness. Perhaps pretty girls have the privilege of keeping their secrets, but the desperate are almost certain to linger in a pool of issues—where abundance and opportunity lie perpetually beyond reach—until they tell all.

That's the most valuable lesson I've learned from the woman with the issue of blood. After all, she'd been dealing with the issue twelve years, an entire spiritual "childhood." And instead of being bettered by her physicians, she was, by this time, quite disillusioned by their inability to heal her. Like the typical natural adolescent, she must have been able to mimic their diagnoses sarcastically, murmur their prescriptions with irritation under her breath before they even finished their thoughts. "I know, I know" she must have thought, inwardly rolling her eyes, as they made one after another hopeless diagnosis. But in her daring press toward Jesus, she makes clear that spiritual adolescence, offers us our first real opportunity at self-definition. It gives us the rare opportunity to tell our own stories, and if we truly desire to be whole, to tell all the truth.

If you've spent any time at all around adolescent girls, you understand how they long to be understood. All said, lengthy conversations at the lockers, the late night talks, the seemingly incessant chatter about one thing or another, and lately, the emailing or text messaging ad infinitum—all are attempts to know truth and be truly known. If we better understood their attempts to reach out for something healing, perhaps we would not judge them so harshly. If I had understood my own adolescence better, I might have reached out sooner to tell all, or at least some, of my own truth.

Instead, an extended childhood held me for some time in any number of "issues." I inherited a rigid set of rules about behavior and an equally inflexible view of God as foreboding and slightly vindictive. Even after committing my life to Christ, it seemed as if everything I'd learned about love and God up until now had only been a cruel lure designed to ensnare me—and now that I was "caught," I felt stuck. Nonetheless, in feeble attempts to curry favor, I set up my own even more extensive system of rules. Admittedly, most of them were mere external measures of my goodness, totally incapable of healing my issues. My horrible misunderstanding of Holiness, of what it meant to have been declared "clean," meant fearfully navigating my natural and spiritual adolescence while carefully attempting to avoid every known spiritual pitfall. You can only imagine how obsessively self-righteous I became. And from that self-imposed restraint eventually came resistance. Regret followed not so long after, and, as was almost inevitable, rebellion.

But mine was not the typical adolescent rebellion. No, my single or most singled-minded act of rebellion was consumption. I might have refused to clean my room, stayed out past curfew with the few pretty friends I had, or been so brazen as to pierce my ears. Instead, I ate. Somehow, eating whatever I liked stood in for all the freedoms I felt myself deprived of. Of course, I wasn't aware of this at the time, but it couldn't be clearer to me than it is now.

Truth be told, reckless consumption does not operate much differently than drug abuse, extensive shopping, or illicit sexual behavior. All have a root in rebellion, a refusal to play by the "real" rules and the consequent construction of a set of false ones. This is, after all, essentially the situation of Satan just before his rebellion and infamous fall. He is the "classic" adolescent—willful, arrogant, insistent on having his own way—ultimately irreverent of authority. But that's another chapter!

The writing of this one represents a sort of spiritual coming of age, a crossing over from childhood, through adolescence, and into maturity. It is not surprising, then, that this was the most difficult chapter to write—and one of the last ones. The most challenging element of taming my appetite is acknowledging real desire. For the longest time, I thought that desire was healing, and that "healing" weighed about 135 pounds. But wholeness? To be entirely truthful. I'm still not sure what it weighs.

Nevertheless, I press. If there was a crowd through which that woman had to press, her wholeness must have come at the height of the business day and amid the rush of so many bodies moving every which way at once. How much like adolescence. And if there was a crowd, there must also have been a confusing din of voices, each competing for her ear. How much more like adolescence. But how much also like that place we long for and, with maturity, press toward. Wholeness comes as we break cultural expectations, refuse the role of the outsider, and deliberately, decisively, take our futures into our own hands, touching and telling Jesus—all the truth. And so, if there is a story to tell, one that makes me whole, I suppose that it's *Fill My Heart*. I hope it inspires your own truth telling and then fills your heart.

## *Food for Thought*

1. What desperate issues have plagued you for a long time? What's the first step toward becoming free?

2. Are there ways in which your weight has made you feel like an outsider? How can you begin to develop genuine relationships as you are healed and made whole of your own issues?

# Kill The Fatted Calf

I have to confess, one of my favorite Bible stories has always been the one about the Prodigal Son but not for the reasons you'd probably imagine. I loved the Father! I mean, wasn't he wonderful? Who couldn't love a Father who, knowing you'd made the worst mistake of your young life, not only loved you anyway, but welcomed you home with an extravagant party! And I identified with the prodigal himself—foolish, impulsive, immature. Cut his face out of the family portrait, insert mine, and *voila*! I know firsthand what it's like to choose hastily and poorly, only to return home expecting shame. And while I also know what it's like to receive almost inconceivable grace, I am even more like the elder brother than the prodigal. I'm sure I'm not the only one. Many of us are like him—never quite certain of our place, and as a result of relationships built on performance, we see food as the measure of whether of not we are accepted.

Food almost invariably marks family celebrations. And in the South, we are especially lavish in the ways we use food to express hospitality. From the simplest to the most extravagant, our social interactions are punctuated with platters of food. It's easy to recall Sunday dinners when we hosted church officials or when we simply dined as a family. "White meat" was synonymous with prestige and power, with preachers and papas. It went to them first, to other adults secondly, and only rarely to children. Perhaps it was then that I initiated the elaborate fantasies of what I would eat when I was "grown." I would have what I wanted and as much of it as I wanted! Now don't misunderstand—there was never any lack of food at our house. In fact, my sister, who is several years above me, insists that I knew the most prosperous times in our family. She remembers, she declares, the days of sandwich-spread-only sandwiches—no meat to be found anywhere! I only remember days of plenty. So where did my sense of emptiness come from? How did I come to conclude that the party that should have been thrown and the calf that should have been killed in my honor actually honored another?

It's probably helpful now to turn to Luke 15. In that Biblical account of the prodigal who returned, the fatted calf is only *one* of the Father's gifts. It represents a sort of first-fruits offering, a way of re-establishing covenant. I understand that it was customary during Biblical times for feasts to accompany the initiation of covenants. Isaac blesses Jacob, and not Esau, over a meal. Esther delivers an entire nation with a banquet as the backdrop. Elijah tests the faith of a widow whose final, meager meal is miraculously transformed into an endless smorgasbord. Jesus sits down to dinner with friends he loves—Mary and Martha—as naturally as he'd accompanied them to the tomb of their brother Lazarus just days earlier to resurrect him. And his parting admonitions to his disciples come during a last supper. More often than not, we mark covenants with the sharing of food.

Even so, my sense is that the least of what the elder brother is disturbed by is the actual calf. I believe the other gifts are of far greater value. As in my own life, however, the "fatted calf" comes easily to stand in as an expression of the whole of what we desire most--acceptance. When the elder son returns from the fields to the sounds of celebration, the servant fails to tell him that his brother has been presented a robe, ring, and shoes—only that a fatted calf has been killed in his honor. How significant, and how like my own reduction of the honorable into the consumable—the sort of it, the amount of it, and so on. Too many times to count, I esteemed the size of a slice of cake, the number of French fries left in the bottom of a bag, or whatever other portion I received as the expression of how much I was thought to be worthy of acceptance. Oblivious to the robe or ring or shoes, to what must have been my parents' numerous other gifts of love—I somehow concentrated all my concern on food.

Luke explains that the Father had divided his substance between the two sons: he divided unto them his living. But failing to recognize the inheritance he'd had all along, the elder brother becomes intensely bitter. I am convinced that the resentment he bottled up must have given him indigestion! He refuses to join the party in his brother's honor. And who's never been there? We can all identify with not having gotten what we wanted, and as a result, having resorted to a concentration on food. That's the essence of emotional eating. But what is far more telling is that because of his misaligned relationship with food, the elder son actually begins to behave like a servant instead of a first born son. He becomes contractual. Like the servant, he seems entirely unmoved by the robe, the ring, or the shoes—all significant, even superior, symbols of favor and restoration. He is only angry that while he has served, he has never been served even a kid, much less a fatted calf. But there wasn't just a misaligned relationship with food here—there was a misaligned relationship with his father.

My relationship with my own father wasn't terribly different. I longed for the sort of affirmation most girls do. I wanted to be told I was pretty and graceful—to be picked up and swung about, celebrated as my father's princess. I found his approval irresistible and so, performance-based acceptance became my norm. It wasn't that I doubted his love—it was just that I believed perfect behavior motivated it. And in every observable way except for my weight, I managed exactly that. I made excellent grades, was never a challenge, excelled at everything I attempted, and secretly expected the high honors I'd won in every other facet of my life to distract him from the fact of my weight. But a fact it was, and one that, not surprisingly, increased sharply at adolescence—the time I most desired his verbal affirmation.

Now to be clear, my father was not an unloving or unkind man. Let's just say his emotional quotient, like many men of his generation, left something to be desired. And that, coupled with my incredible sensitivity to even the hint of disapproval was enough. And so, while I longed for his affirmation of my beauty and acceptability, I grudgingly swallowed his praise of my academic performance. That, at least, was constant. But performance-based relationships are inherently unstable. Like the elder brother of the prodigal, I might have realized that I already had access to my father's heart if I hadn't so desperately needed what seemed impossible to have.

But unhealthy family relationships often cause us to give food a more significant role than it should have. And so what I could have, I decided, was food. Whether we eat too much because we're hard pressed to say what's really on our minds or associate food with love so that we give the former in more abundance than the latter, we are probably misusing food. If we see the delineations between our siblings and ourselves in terms of portions or if we are using food as a representation of acceptance, we are likely to be missing the real gifts of love our families can give. Most importantly, we are likely to be missing the gifts that God himself desires to give.

You see, I am more and more convinced of the simplicity of the faith message. I may take issue with the faith movement, per se, but I am completely convinced of the faith message because it is, quite simply, that there is more than enough. Whatever the need, there is more than enough. What tends to happen when we are consumed by food as the expression of "enough," though, is that it immediately begins to shrink. Whether what we need is literally food or money or relationship, it shrinks when we see it in isolation from all that it is possible to receive.

I have a dear friend who is a culinary whiz! Her forte' is not so much cooking well, though she does. It is that she has hit on an impeccable truth: good food in and of itself does not produce a fine dining experience. Fine dining necessarily entails good friends, a soothing atmosphere, a beautiful setting and a table at which one is accepted for the gifts she brings. My friend understands that fatted calves alone do not make for celebration. Rather, the robe, the ring, the shoes, the Father—these are what make the party!

This was clearly the case in Biblical cultures, where the robe was one sign of authority and favor. Joseph's coat of many colors was his father's indication that he was more loved than his brothers. And so it might have been that the elder brother in Luke 15 was understandably offended at his father's extravagant display of affection. And when he offered the ring as additional evidence of his approval, as it was often a symbol of influence and belonging, even the best of us can understand how the elder brother must have felt justified in his bitterness, right? I mean, when a king sent an emissary forth to speak on his behalf, he sent him with a signet ring. That ring could be used as a seal every bit as legitimate as our modern day signatures. But the shoe must have taken the brother over the edge! You'll recall, no doubt, that the removal and giving of one's shoe was a gesture that sealed a Biblical covenant. If not, check out the story of Ruth again, where Boaz seals her selection as his wife by giving the nearer kinsman his shoe. I cannot say with certainty what the father intended in giving these gifts, other than unconditional forgiveness. But I certainly cannot dismiss the elder son's response. It hurts to see another preferred above oneself when the sole measure of love is what can be consumed.

But when the measure of love is productive—when its potency is determined by how much life it gives—that is another matter altogether. The father's sole reason for lavishing any of his gifts upon the son who, admittedly and already acknowledges his unworthiness, is that he has come back to life! He has come back to himself. He had, the prior verses explain, been longing to fill himself with the husks fed to swine. That word longing means "to set the heart upon." He was hungry for more than food. He was hungry for home.

There are any number of reasons why food becomes the primary, if not single way we express our love in our families. Perhaps the most compelling of them is that it is such a primal representation of need and of sustenance. But if we're ever to understand the other gifts family brings, and those we desperately need to receive, we'll have to surpass the need to live on bread alone. We'll have to wrap up in robes that warm our spirits, put on rings that serve as simple reminders of whose we are, and this time, on holy ground, put our shoes back on. Finally, we can come home.

## Food for Thought

1. Have you ever used food as a measure of acceptance, or love even, in your own family? If so, what was the real source of frustration that consumption masked?

2. Perhaps your family's "fatted calf" wasn't food, but something else. In any case, if you ever felt less honored/honorable than another member of your family, ask God now to help you to forgive. Now, what practical steps can be taken to mend the relationship?

# *Naked and Ashamed*

It would be impossible and impractical to write a book about weight and not deal with the very painful issues surrounding rejection, particularly by men. And since they are where most of my rejection issues originated, I must. Two divorces and countless badly chosen relationships (not to speak of the ones that "chose" me) required that I confront the relation between generational patterns, childhood trauma, unhealthy relationships and weight. All have acted like a sort of spiritual and emotional shrapnel, entering via a single wound, but breaking up and creating various sorts of internal chaos. I could as easily be writing about the implications of weight in my spending since overspending, like overeating, often masks real need. Or I could have written of a jaded sexual identity, not so much in terms of numbers of relationships, but certainly in terms of grossly misconstrued notions of Godly sexuality since misguided sexuality, like overeating, always masks a desire for real intimacy. I am deliberately focusing on weight because, for me, it has acted as the fulcrum on which the others balance.

As self-revelation after self-revelation occurred during the writing of this book, I found particular and necessary comfort in simple scriptures. One of them was Romans 8:1-2: "There is therefore now no condemnation to them which are in Christ Jesus, who walk not after the flesh, but after the Spirit. For the law of the Spirit of life in Christ Jesus hath made me free from the law of sin and death." I might not have been able to complete this chapter without that assurance. Sin always invokes a penalty, whether for the sinner or the one sinned against. When we sin, the penalty can be immediate and obvious or take years to surface. Likewise, when someone sins against us, we may experience either immediate or remote implications, if not both. Either way, unresolved sin tends to lead to shame.

Shame: It's the root of my struggle with weight. In truth, shame is at the root of most of the struggles we experience. It was at the center of Adam's and Eve's refusal to return to God after the Fall and, ever since, has been asserting its influence over our thoughts about ourselves and God. When Adam and Eve fell, they experienced a traumatic rending of relationship, a rejection of sorts, and the impact was shame. The Bible explains that, without any apparent external motivation to do so, they hid themselves. They understood implicitly that sin had somehow "uncovered" them and immediately attempted to cover themselves.

While rejection produces any number of effects, shame is the primary one. Shame feeds off of fear, and fear prevents real intimacy. It inevitably leads us to hide and, from our crouching position just behind whatever the closest "fig bush" might be, we emerge bitter and angry. Shame can cause us to blame as Adam blamed Eve, and as Eve blamed the serpent. But shame also encourages and validates a level of irresponsibility that, while it has public implications, mostly eats away at us inwardly. That kind of inward emptiness keeps us from being honest with ourselves and leads to insincerity and superficiality—further guards against true intimacy.

I can say those things because I know all too well how shame caused me to cover myself. The most obvious "cover" of course, is weight. But shame did not simply cause me to hide my body. It often caused me to hide my better self. Every emotion, every response, and every thought was carefully considered and critiqued. And until "approved," all were contained—until I started to lose weight. In fact, it was a crisis of realization that I was becoming less and less of myself that initiated lasting weight loss. Through a series of traumas I barely acknowledged—a miscarriage, death, divorce, dreams lost—I had gradually given up more and more of myself, telling less and less truth, and fearing rejection if I somehow managed to say or do something authentic. I covered my self emotionally and spiritually, much as I'd covered myself physically to protect against further trauma. What I have recently begun to understand is that those adult traumas could not be separated from and, indeed, had to be understood in the light of God's truth about past ones.

As I began to write this book, the Lord began to deal seriously with my shame, connecting generational patterns and childhood traumas to adult reiterations of the same. Somewhere around the time I was 10, whether as an adolescent prank or with more harmful intent, my brother exposed himself to me. That was the extent of the violation, but for years, I could not acknowledge that it had even occurred. I was overwhelmed by terrific fear and, of course, the sort of shame that surrounds children who think that, in some way they've contributed to whatever bad there is in their worlds. The exposure troubled me not simply as an emotional and sexual violation; it hurt me most because it wrestled from me the only man, aside from my father, who might have affirmed me then. As a result, most of my relationships with men have been about recovering that affirmation. With little consciousness of my behavior, even less of my intent, I sought approval, acceptance, affirmation, acknowledgement…the list goes on. Sometimes I seemed to get it. Most times I did not, and when I did not, I attributed their rejection to my weight. It became the single lens—skewed as it was—through which I would see all rejection.

In some ways, it might not seem like such a false starting place. After all, we are so thoroughly culturally conditioned on standards of beauty that we're hardly aware of any distinctions between what we honestly prefer and what we are told we should prefer through various media. Much has been made of advertisements aimed at women and young girls designed to condition us to assess ourselves, mostly negatively, and always comparatively.

Even more might be made of the impact of those advertisements on men. But assessments of advertising are largely a matter of the mind. Rejection is always, at last, a matter of the heart. Studies and findings aside, realizations reached and adaptations made, we deal with rejection emotionally. As I said at the outset of this chapter, rejection may lead to many sorts of excess. It is always in search of one thing, however, and that is fullness.

The most obvious sort of fullness, of course, is physical. Emotional eating literally kept me from feeling. But rejection caused me to create an even less obvious, and therefore more dangerous, sort of fullness—distance. As a child, I loved bubbles—still do! Their resilience fascinates me. Washing dishes recently, I noticed this one bubble across the top of a glass. I placed a spoon in the glass—the bubble was unharmed. I thought, surely a fork will pierce it, but its tines were as easily received as the spoon. Nearly invisible, a bubble is a most durable thing. It will not break until the pressure within it exceeds the pressure outside of it.

Imagine if you will yourself within a bubble. You can see out and others can see in but only from a distance. They can approach, but they are never able to touch you because of the bubble. The bubble is elastic, so it takes its dimensions from the situation. If you need more distance, the bubble increases and allows for that. But even if it shrinks, the bubble is absolutely unyielding and will not let others in—unless the pressure within exceeds the pressure without.

The emotional distance or "bubble" I built between my brother and me eventually expanded to others. The discomfort and detachment I felt around him was magnified until it created a whole culture of secrecy and isolation. I made small attempts to express my fears—once in a suggestive drawing—but mostly I kept silent and ate. When my brother was punished once for calling me fat, I could not even celebrate his humiliation. He was made to "apologize" by repeating that very insult about himself. But even as he broke down in tears, more in shame than repentance, I did not celebrate. Perhaps it was compassion that made me cry with him. More likely, I had internalized the lessons of rejection. I could only celebrate if

I was willing to account for my triumph. But since I was not able to celebrate the ultimate victory over his violation, the fat thing seemed a trivial matter. Triumph only comes when the pressure from within exceeds the pressure from without. I could find no words of judgment, however, no "good for you" that surpassed my shame, so I kept silent and ate. And while I did not express typical anger then in verbal backlash, acting out, or rebellion—I was every bit as angry as Eve, having realized her nakedness and every bit as inept as she was at covering her shame.

As unable as she had been to name my real enemy, I blamed everything on fat and blamed fat for everything. Every missed opportunity or ruined relationship somehow wound down to that. And while weight may have been partly to blame, I never stopped to account for any greater relational weaknesses I might have addressed. As if that were not enough, my anger caused me to become aloof. If an unwary walk down the hallway had resulted in my seeing what I never should have, I would be even less engaged, particularly when it came to men—more cautious. I would never be caught off guard again by a half-opened bedroom door. I would make myself completely impenetrable to trauma. I would not make eye-contact or, God forbid, smile at them. And I most certainly would not feel.

Of course, these were not absolute rules. I did risk exposure and love. Still, it always seemed like more of a risk than some liberating release of control. When I did love, it was seldom with the sort of abandon I imagined to be the privilege those who'd never internalized rejection. I can only say that years of counsel and continuous deliverance are increasing the pressure within the bubble! Shortly before losing my brother to cancer, I forgave him totally. We were at our parents' flower shop in North Carolina. Alone in the front display room, and just before he set out with one of the day's deliveries, I simply said "I forgive you." He looked at me quizzically, genuine innocence reflected in his eyes. He seemed altogether unable to imagine why I would need to forgive him and seemed to struggle with this small gesture of intimacy, but I knew that I was piercing years of shame and silence—breaking out naked and completely unashamed.

Months later, I gave his eulogy, but not before a sequence of cards and conversations about and, of course, prayers for his salvation. Just shy of 40 years, many of them plagued by his own struggles and early rejections, no doubt, he died. I'm relieved that he was not hungry for forgiveness.

## Food for Thought

1. Are any of your eating habits connected to shame? Secrecy? If so, what are the real roots of that shame?

2. If you've experienced traumatic childhood events, you may want help dealing with them. Commit today to sharing with one trusted friend where your heart has been wounded and ask for help seeking healing.

# Tried in the Balance...and Found "Wanting"

I owe whatever success I can claim in the area of weight management and healthy living to so many people that it's hard to know where to begin my acknowledgments. I might begin with all the people who, with good intentions I'm sure, commented favorably whenever I began to lose weight. Never mind that their eventual silence quietly but conversely marked its return. I hardly needed a scale. I had only to listen to the commentary of others to know how I appeared to be doing. And I would be remiss if I did not acknowledge those who thought my face "so pretty," as if it existed all on its own, detached entirely from my body. And sometimes it seemed so—or I made it seem so. For whatever my body was feeling, I was usually quite adept at hiding it with my face. In the course of so many years, one learns to smile—particularly in the quiet moments. You might have expected that I'd have begun any real acknowledgements with God. And I might have, since he has been such an impeccable model of unconditional love to me that I would be foolish to start anywhere else.

But the truth is, I've spent far too much of my life in pursuit of ungodly acknowledgment than in real affirmation. And since acknowledgment is external, and comes from others, it has been the location of many of my struggles with self esteem. Until recently, though, I don't think I even knew the difference. Acknowledgment is the recognition of another's existence, validity, authority, or right. As it suggests, it stems from a word having to do with knowledge, specifically knowledge of another other than oneself. Affirmation, on the other hand, is an entirely different sort of declaration. It is simply the declaration that something is true. It need not come from without. In fact, it seldom does.

But if we are unaware of this subtle distinction, and if we are mostly accustomed to outward measures of our progress, we will always find ourselves "wanting," that is, lacking in some way. Whether those outward measures be the sorts of positive acknowledgement that, in moments of sudden silence, can leave us feeling worth-less and unbalanced—or the literal scales on which we delicately balance hope and reality, we can find ourselves "wanting," hoping to measure up to some exterior standard that, even when met, fails to genuinely affirm.

That was the case with two brothers—Jacob and Esau. Dramatically different even before birth, each was loved by one parent, neither by both. Jacob, we are told, is loved by Rebekah— just because. And Esau is loved by Isaac, mostly because of his performance. He is loved because of what he can produce and what he can produce is food. As the well-known story goes, he trades his birthright because of his own appetite, and eventually, because of his father's, loses his blessing as well. He is his father's son. But their similarity does not begin and end with appetite. Esau so easily disregards his birthright because he believes he's about to die of hunger. Isaac, clearly suspicious of the circumstances under which he's getting the very thing he asked for, nonetheless disregards his "gut" feeling and fulfills his appetite. Feeling himself close to death, he becomes undiscerning.

What's to be learned here about the nature of rejection? Well, the first thing is that is often sets us up for a lifetime of running. Scarred by some original pain, we often leave home trying desperately to outrun the source of that pain. And when we finally meet up with it again, we usually find out that we could have confronted and forgiven it long ago. But there's another lesson as well. Early rejections, denials of elemental need, often set us up to over-react to future denials. What would it have cost Esau to wait? What would it have cost him to keep his birthright and his appetite in check? And there's another thing to reckon with here; early rejections can often set us up to overestimate the power of future ones. We remain in failing relationships, we cling to dysfunctional patterns, we profess our love time and again for what looks like a new lover only to realize that we have chosen the old one again. Early rejections can create such a sense of hopelessness that, at the slightest provocation—hunger—we feel that we will perish. And so we eat.

To be sure, I've spanned the range of possibility when it came to scales. I've refused to weigh at all, but then again, I've weighed daily or even more often—sometimes before and after exercise, or a meal, or a trip to the bathroom. I've compared scales—my doctor's, the gym's, the scale I keep near the refrigerator—anything to be sure I was meeting the mark. And I confess, I've even risked quarters to rest stop restroom scales, not to mention the insult and injury of the "fortune for the day," just to know if I'd lost weight between states. Clearly, I've been obsessed with measures.

And so, I know what it feels like to succeed or seemingly fail on the basis of any number of factors influencing weight—none of them related to healthy behavior. It's clear that even from my scale, I've mostly been in search of acknowledgement.

But my appetite for truth is becoming insatiable. And so, now that I'm thinking deliberately of just what the ideal "measure" might be, and even knowing that perfection is an impossible dream, I'm amazed at how much I've tried to measure up—mostly by erasing as much singularity as I could. Monochromatic worked on so many levels, not the least of which is dress. If everything at least seemed to "blend," I thought, there were bound to be fewer points at which I must reckon with what does not fit or what does not flow. Monochromatic clothing, I thought, at least permitted me refuge from lines that refused to, well, fall in line, as they were actually unruly bulges here and there. Past clothing choices, in my desire for acknowledgement, I sought outward conformity through adherence to as normal a standard as I could make myself observe. My highest aim became a bland and inoffensive spirit. I've hoped that by blending in emotionally, I could draw less attention to myself and that by doing so, I could ultimately arrive at invisibility.

Only now do I realize that invisibility is as far as one can get from affirmation. Fairly well, I had mastered the art of hiding from others—but where could I hide from myself? And even more to the point, where could I ever even attempt to hide from God? Even when I ran from Him, resisted Him, rebelled outright—He affirmed me. He never stopped speaking truth about me—and that was the deepest desire of my heart—to know the truth about myself. How well, how intimately I understood Psalm 51—as if it were a mirror image of myself, for I was ever before myself. I could not escape.

From all of the years of wrestling and unrest, of weariness or outright disgust with my body, it seemed I could not escape. I was always "before" myself. In other words, even I was only capable of acknowledgment, not affirmation. I could only think or speak of myself in terms of what an outsider might see. And like an outsider, I only approved myself when I was meeting some external measure. Or if I could not approve, I was pretending to.

And so, because it created a kind of distance between myself and, well, my self, I lived with a rather schizophrenic self image. I was only acceptable, or worthy of love, or deserving of the affirmation that I had confused with acknowledgment, if I measured up by exterior scales. What I meant, and what most of us mean when we say we've suffered from low self-esteem is just that: we have held up the mirror of exterior acknowledgment expecting interior affirmation. As if before the famous mirror in a well-known fairy tale, even we have—from time to time at least—been told that we are "fair." Once the exterior acknowledgment ceases, however, we become cruel and vengeful.

But the truth is that acknowledgement never suffices for affirmation, even if there seems to be a steady flow of it. And while it is true that others may see and acknowledge what we have ourselves found to be true, affirmation always comes first.

I could tell you that I make a point of lingering in the mirror, of telling myself from time to time that I am beautiful. I do not, and perhaps I should. What I can say now, however, is that I no longer fear the mirror's response, and should it ever tell me that there are others fairer than I, I will simply smile—genuinely this time. It was this way, I imagine, when Esau met up again with Jacob. Without one thought of retaliation, he embraces him, even while refusing his offerings and "Keep what you have; I have more than enough." I'd call that fullness!

## Food for Thought

1. Other than pounds lost on a scale, what could one measure of your "success" be in this area?

2. How has the assessment of others either helped or hindered your self-image?

# I Came for Form—and If I Can Manage It—Fashion

If you had the privilege of growing into your sense of self amidst those grand church ladies I spoke of earlier, you already recognize the singularly ironic catch phrase from every seriously spiritual sister's testimony: "I didn't come here for form or fashion. I didn't come to see or be seen!" Those were fighting words! Hats might get shouted on. Wigs could fly off or at very least sit twisted on the wearer's head after a good, hearty praise! Most certainly, half-slips were going to sag once The Spirit took over. Once a woman declared war on "form and fashion," it was on!

I suppose the irony lay in this: no one took more precious care in covering their bodies as elegantly as these very sisters. Sometimes, elegance meant opulence. Sequins and lace and matching hats, shoes, purses, not to mention handkerchiefs—well, those were understood to be standard church fare. But even the more modest, the "sweetly saved" in their sanctified "to the ankle" skirts were as carefully attentive to cover themselves. Don't get me wrong, I'm all for genuine modesty. I think what I've only recently come to resist is the way that our "church clothes" obscured other, far more problematic matters than an exposed elbow or ankle. Those church clothes hid a multitude of bumps and bulges and rolls and, well, I'll just say it—fat.

I have tried not to make this book explicitly religious in nature. As a matter of fact, I owe a great deal of its delay to religion. Religion maintains the status quo—spiritual, emotional, even physical—by covering truth, and if there's anything I mean to accomplish here, its exposure. And so, I almost called this chapter *Taking off My Church Clothes: Laying Aside the Weight of Religiosity*, but it sounded a bit too pompous—too mocking. After all, I owe most of the good that survived the (mis)adventures of my life to women of terrific strength and character, church women who taught me to honor God. Even so, as I strip away the habit of hiding behind an unwieldy set of expectations about dress—weighty in their own right—I am struck by the degree to which church clothes accomplished radically different, dual ends.

Of course, we looked the best we looked all week on Sundays. And why shouldn't we have? For many, the only really important person we were going to meet all week was God! And furthermore, it was the most important we were going to be all week—meeting Him. But looking our best most often meant hiding our flaws, putting on layer after layer of clothing meant to "shield" others from temptation, but which in all reality, helped hold us in denial about how bad a shape we were in—literally.

Clothing can be something of a refuge it's true, but when the naked truth—pun absolutely intended—is that one's nakedness cannot be hidden, either physically or spiritually, not even by clothing, a confrontation is inevitable. Most of us see clothing as an expression of who we are. If we did not, we would not spend thousands of dollars on it annually, and we would not make such painstaking attempts to coordinate and accentuate and accessorize. We dress as we do for approval—for acknowledgment. If we did not, we might never change. We might not change our church clothes, and we might not change our bodies. But change is exactly what our bodies and spirits are craving if we have challenges with weight. Clothing seems to set before us constant opportunities to create and recreate our images until we arrive at one or two that reflect how we want to see and be seen.

But when we are naked, only one of two things is possible. We may either see ourselves as having been created in the image of God, or we can see ourselves as somehow far less than that perfect (and perhaps false) image we carry of Adam and Eve. Of course, I know that Genesis is speaking as much of spiritual purity as of physical nakedness, but "bare" with me for a moment. ☺ If they were, after all, naked and not ashamed, was it because they'd have met today's model-perfect standards of beauty? And since many of us who do not meet that standard are left naked and so obviously ashamed, we presume that we could not possibly have been created as they were—perfect, entire, lacking nothing.

And so begins our quest to complete the imperfect, to perfect the incomplete. And what a mess we've made of it. In our efforts to contribute something, anything, exterior to that which is lacking, to fill up what often remains a dangerous and desperate void, we have simply hidden behind layer after layer of church clothes. And I don't simply mean materially, I mean spiritually.

What if we couldn't hide in them—behind them? What if instead of the sequins and lace, the furs and matching accessories of every sort—what if the simple linen robe of the Old Testament priest was our common attire? And I don't even mean the exterior robes worn for public worship. I mean that barest of robes—the one reserved for the most private worship in the most holy place. What if, instead of concealing us, our church clothes truly exposed us, to ourselves and to God? Then it might be possible to express both form and fashion. After all, we were formed, made, and fashioned by God's awesome design—and out from under a few of our church clothes—we might just learn to love the image He's given us. Now I'd call that the height of fashion!

## *Food for Thought*

1. How have clothes enhanced either your positive self-image or your self-consciousness? How much should they do either?

2. Consider the conventions of dress at the church you attend. Consider what the style of dress suggests about the place, people, experience…

# Hide Me:
# Developing the Lifestyle of Weightless Worship

There are a great many things we'll do for love that we will not do for any other cause. When love is pure, there is hardly anything more powerful. But when love is corrupted by unrighteous desire, it becomes the single most potentially destructive power we can know.

Lucifer's story has always amazed me for that reason. In my best moments, I soberly ponder what would cause one to forfeit the incredible opportunity to worship before the throne of God. What could possibly be more fulfilling than that? Like Adam and Eve, Lucifer had no earthly complaint against God. He was beautifully created, arrayed in every imaginable jewel. He was wise, and increased his wealth because of that wisdom. And his talents perfectly matched his assignment—worship. Where is it said that when he merely moved, he made music? That is the model of worship—and the model of integrity. We were created to *be* what we were assigned to *do*—in that order. But when things become disordered, when we begin to do without first being, we can become self-destructive. Ezekiel says it best: speaking of the King of Tyre and some would say of Lucifer, he says "you had the seal of perfection," that is to say, you were the model or pattern, the original of worship—until your beauty became deceptive.

If the original vision of worship was that it be a seamless melding of inside and out, an unwavering devotion to God that, in its realization, made us more beautiful and brilliant—that's the sort of worship I want to give to God! That's the essence of pure worship. It has so much less to do with singing or dancing, so little to do with performance of any sort. Too often, though, I think we've made the mistake of measuring God's intent by the "fallen" creation. We measure ourselves among ourselves, invariably coming up wanting, because we've never received a fully developed picture of what God envisioned for us in creation. We struggle with false images and ideologies of worship, and not inconsequentially, with images of beauty, mostly because we've never seen an accurate description of the way He sees us. We should not be surprised, then, when the picture we carry of ourselves is grossly distorted in every other place than pure worship.

I hardly feel the impact of weight in worship. My voice takes me places, at the leading of the Spirit, that my body is compelled to keep up with. I don't say that to suggest that there aren't consequences to weight, even when I am most about my Father's business and most immersed in purpose. But if there is anywhere that I feel almost weightless, it is in His presence.

One of my favorite Psalms has become 91. It speaks of hiddenness, of secrecy and shadows. And I admit that before I found my way in worship, those had an entirely different significance to me. Throughout much of my adolescence, I seldom made eye contact with anyone. Even in the safety of church, my most vivid recollections are of shoes. When I shook hands I saw, not faces, but feet. Even when I began more public music ministry, I refused to wear my glasses. Absent them, I could look out into an audience and not see. And if I could not see, I could not be seen. You see, singing is not at all the same as worshipping. Singing is performance, and performance provides a cloak of anonymity. It is a perfect vocation for those who would hide. And so, for most of my growing-up years, I sang. For many of my adult years, I sang. I led choirs and assembled ensembles, but I never worshipped, that is to say, I was never lost to myself, completely unconscious of my body or careless about how it might appear to others, until recently.

The thing about worship is that, once you've ever experienced the weightlessness of it, the absolute freedom of it, you can never go back to singing. It can be inconvenient, though, because at times we all want to hide. We want not to be vulnerable or transparent. Even with God, we sometimes want to preserve ourselves from the intent and intentional gaze that, somewhere deep inside, we suspect will deliver censure.

But worship is the practice of transparency. And so, at some of my most difficult moments, my songs have reflected that difficulty. They were songs of experience or if they were worship songs, they were sung with more consciousness of what I was experiencing than expecting. What I am only now coming to understand is that the songs were never meant to hide the experiences. Worship was meant to convey the best and worst of us to God. We have some faulty notion that true worship is flawless—and in one sense it is. It is flawless in its admiration and affirmation of who God is. And in its essence, it reflects none of us. But in its conveyance—the means by which we deliver what we've surrendered—it is shaped in every way by who we are.

I am a firm believer that, even as the Bible clearly reveals, we are three part beings—spirit, soul, and body. I think we'd mostly agree to that, but as for the relation between the three, the delicate balance that God has always intended—we're far from agreement on what that looks like. In an attempt to achieve sinless perfection, we have disregarded, disdained even, the body as anything more than a shell. And while it is undeniable that the greatest part of who we are is spirit—one has to wonder why, if the body were to be ignored, God put it there at all. If it was even the case with Lucifer, that the outside is meant in some way to permit a glimpse at the inside, we have to start acknowledging the importance of reaching a healthy weight. In that lies a profound key to our health, not only body by body, but as the Body of Christ.

Throughout this book, I have attempted to focus as broadly as a mostly autobiographical work would allow me to. I have told my stories, engaging at times, I hope, with yours. And if you happen not to be a Christian, I think you'll identify with much of the truth I've told anyway.

But if you are a Christian, I imagine you've had an entirely different experience of this book—and now—you have an entirely different mandate. Romans 8 puts it this way:

> For the anxious longing of the creation waits eagerly for the revealing of the sons of God. For the creation was subjected to futility, not willingly, but because of Him who subjected it, in hope that the creation itself also will be set free from its slavery to corruption into the freedom of the glory of the children of God. For we know that the whole creation groans and suffers the pains of childbirth together until now. And not only this, but also we ourselves, having the first fruits of the Spirit, even we ourselves groan within ourselves, waiting eagerly for our adoption as sons, the redemption of our body.

Allow me to paraphrase and elaborate. They're waiting for us! Not so much for the next great diet—but for the perfection of the balance that was in the beginning and which has been missing ever since. The world has been waiting, not for one more crafty means of tricking the body into some unnatural process of elimination. That is the futility to which we have been submitted. And if we are ever to be set free from that futility, it will be by hope. It's my deepest wish that this book has inspired that. That while it sometimes dealt with difficult and painful realities, it also inspired the sort of hope that has the capacity to set us free from corruption and set us on the road to redemption.

*Hide Me: Developing the Lifestyle of Weightless Worship*

I'm convinced now more than ever that the shift from a local to a global mindset is the key to any significant change. My desire and now my need to lose weight hangs on that. It is not simply that I expect my own life to change, but that I anticipate having an impact on the body of Christ, on the nations of the world, and on the coming of the Kingdom.

As I concluded the writing of this book, I began to see a glimpse of opportunity and realize even more of an obligation. So much is waiting! As I said at the outset, this book only represents a beginning. Health is a journey that requires attention, day by day, pound by pound. And I should know—I've started and stopped too many diets to count. The single difference now is that I am committed to more than myself. I have seen just a glimpse of my Kingdom design and that, I pray, is more than enough to fuel the next steps and to continue to fill my heart.

It won't always be easy, but it will be an honest process as pure worship disarms and disrobes us. It puts us utterly at ease in the presence of God who, since we are only present to acknowledge and adore Him, radiates his pleasure and approval back as we do so. No small wonder, I am capable of movement in worship that I would otherwise never even attempt. I dance, less conscious of myself than at any other moment, because in pure worship, I am weightless.

And it's not just that I feel physically lighter, though that is true. It's that in no other place with God do I so clearly understand his design for me. Face to face with Him, I so totally understand my worth. And the fact that worship isn't about me doesn't phase God one bit! He delights so much in pure worship that it blesses him to reaffirm us there. So if you've struggled as I have with body image or self esteem, I encourage you to throw your hands up—in literal and spiritual abandon. I encourage you to find just one place where you can sing at the top of your lungs! Where you can dance wildly and passionately! Find a place where you can be weightless in worship!

In that place God will affirm who He is and who you are, only because of His love. You see, more than we realize, worship has reciprocal effects. What Lucifer failed to understand is that he need not have declared his right to "ascend" to any height. In pure worship, there is absolutely no need to make ourselves bigger or smaller than we are. We only need to be.

When God gave you the body He gave you, He already had your Kingdom purpose in mind. He ultimately wants worship and worshippers who reflect His glory in every way. And so, Lucifer's beauty and brilliance wasn't for his own ascent, it was to be for the glory of God. Likewise, it's true that your body was made as an invitation to the Spirit of God, a habitation. And if He can be comfortable in it, so can you! Think about it: when God selected you for His purposes, it was as if He was choosing a house. If you've ever done that, you know what I mean. You see every space as yours potentially. You imagine your favorite things in just the right places, and you envision your personality and flair being expressed in every room. You may initially be drawn to the neighborhood or even to the exterior of the house, but you dream of living inside it! That's exactly the way God thinks of you—He dreams of living in you!

If you've read this book without ever having personally experienced a relationship with God through His son Jesus Christ, I encourage you to commit to Him now. He will take the weight of sin from you and change your life forever! Even If you have a relationship with Christ, but have never known the liberty that comes from weightless worship, I encourage you to put this book down now and, well, do whatever worship looks like to you! Sing your freest song! Dance your wildest dance! Write your most expressive poem! Let your heart be filled with the hope that God knows your, er, His address—your heart! Let Him live in every bit of it today and fill it completely!

## Food for Thought

1. What have you learned about yourself as you read this book?

2. What's next? What areas of change have you discovered, and how can you begin to move toward practical change?

# 12

# Sweeter Than Honey: Prayers to Pray Along the Way

## To Receive Jesus Christ as Savior

Heavenly Father,

I realize that what I've hungered for more than anything is the certainty of relationship with you through your son, Jesus Christ. I confess my sin now, accept his forgiveness, and ask you to release me from every one of my old ways. Make me the new creation you promise I can be through Jesus Christ.

## To Receive the Holy Spirit

Heavenly Father,

In relationship with you I've found more peace and joy than I'd ever imagined possible. Thank you! My hunger to be completely filled with your Spirit, to be led, taught and comforted by Him is my heart's desire. Father, you promised to satisfy with good things those who ask in faith. So, I ask you now for the presence and power of your Spirit to fill me completely. As they do, to transform me into the powerful carrier of your purpose in the earth through Jesus Christ.

## Healing From Rejection

Heavenly Father,

Teach me what it really means to be accepted in the beloved—you! Mend my heart and show me what it looks like to approach the mirror—not just the natural one, but the one of your word—and love what I see. Thank you for releasing me from the fear of failure to please others. Now Father, completely fill me with the desire to reflect only your glory through Jesus Christ.

## Forgiveness of Those Who've Inflicted Pain

Heavenly Father,

Because you've forgiven me, I can forgive others. I choose to forgive and release all who've hurt me—intentionally or not—with painful words and actions. In doing so, I pray that you make us both (all) free to love in the way that Jesus Christ loved even those who rejected him. Remove every trace of the pain that used to be and, if there are scars of any sort, Father, may they only remind me of the healing that has already taken place by the blood of Jesus Christ.

## Healing from Self-Rejection

Heavenly Father,

I've sometimes just not "been there" for myself, and now I ask you not only to forgive me but to strengthen me against self-pity, self-rejection, self-sabotage. Make me bold, even as you keep me vulnerable. Make me a delight to myself, even as you increase genuine humility. Cause me to rise up like the champion I am — and cheer myself on to victory! I encourage myself in you so that I can encourage others. I love the fearfully, wonderfully made miracle you are causing me to become through Jesus Christ!

## Physical Healing

Heavenly Father,

This temple sometimes aches with the literal weight it has held up. Even as you're releasing me day by day from the physical limitations that once held me, release the spirit of praise where heaviness used to overwhelm and impede me. Enable me to walk, run, or soar — to simply accomplish my measure — with the courage of the eagle. And Father, at every new physical challenge, cause me to embrace your ability in me. I really can do all things through Christ who strengthens, and heals, and renews me!

## Deliverance and Healing from Anorexia/Bulimia

Heavenly Father,

I acknowledge my desperation for you. I realize that the struggles I have are not with flesh and blood, but with spiritual powers for whom I am no match on my own. My only hope for victory is your strength. You are more than a match for anything I come up against! There is no power that can prevail against yours, Father. Thank you for releasing me from every work of my enemy and for, day by day, creating in me a new heart. Cause me to see what you see, and to see as you see through Jesus Christ.

## Prayer for New Appetite(s)

Heavenly Father,

Thank you for training me in your ways and for increasing my spiritual and natural stamina so that I consistently choose what is best. Father, I admit that I don't always prefer what is best, and in those times, I most need you to remind me of your strength at work in me. Teach me how to retrain every one of my affections and appetites so that I fuel my body not simply to please my tastes, but to fulfill my purpose in the earth through Jesus Christ.

## Freedom to Embrace a New Image

Heavenly Father,

I am surrounded by so many voices—all of them shouting what I should be, none of them yours. Help me to be still and know you. As your voice stills me, Father, I will be able to know the difference between the truth and a lie. And once I know the truth, Father, I'm free to reject unhealthy media images in pursuit of your vision of who I am indeed. Even as my body changes for the better, help me to see, acknowledge and affirm the changes! And Father, when I do not see all that I expect, remind me of the tremendous work going on, as you fill my heart!

# *Endorsement*

The heartbeat of this book comes from the inward cry of a woman who so exquisitely expounds on a personal and sensitive, yet much needed topic, "fat." Please don't be deceived by the word "fat," as the contents of this book far exceed the matter of being overweight or obese. The author shares her real-life, heartfelt experiences along with familiar Biblical stories, challenging us to see how "fat" has infiltrated our lives, through various appetites other than food, yet leaving us still hungry and unfilled. I have been truly inspired to re-evaluate my own thinking towards my greatest struggle--"obesity," as I have received great revelation from this soul-searching book. I commend the author for her openness and transparency to face the whole truth.

*Susan J. Ridley*

Playwright and Author

www.ingramcontent.com/pod-product-compliance
Lightning Source LLC
Chambersburg PA
CBHW031300290426
44109CB00012B/658